LIVING WITH
ADDISON'S DISEASE

*A Guide for People with Addison's,
Supporters and Professionals*

Professor **Simon Pearce**

Sarah Spain

Living with Addison's Disease – A Guide for People with Addison's, Supporters and Professionals

Copyright © 2019 Addison's Disease Self-Help Group

Authors :
      Professor Simon HS Pearce
      Sarah Spain

With contributions from :
      Professor John Wass
      Dr Victoria Rouse
      Dr Tim Cheetham
      Phillip Yeoh
      Neil McClements
      Hannah Kerr-Peterson
      Lincoln Tsang

This edition was first published with ❤ in the United Kingdom by the Addison's Disease Self-Help Group, a registered charity/non-profit with the Charity Commission for England & Wales (registration number 1179825). We work to support people affected by Addison's disease. Join us at www.addisonsdisease.org.uk. Together, we are stronger.

A CIP catalogue record for this book is available from the British Library

ISBN 978-1-5272-3664-6

Table of Contents

04

What Kind of Quality of Life Can I Expect?   41

Foreword

Friends,

It seems like only yesterday that I founded the Addison's Disease Self-Help Group on my dining room table in 1984.

When the group started, it was all about self-help. Addison's remains a rare endocrine condition, which is often poorly understood, despite the best efforts of the medical community.

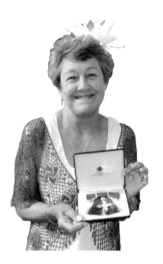

And so it's vital that as people affected by Addison's (or caring for others with the condition), we get educated and learn how to manage it for ourselves.

So, I'm delighted to introduce you to this book! It's a valuable resource for us all, as we learn to thrive, not just survive, on our daily journey with Addison's disease. I wish I'd had a copy when I was first diagnosed...

Over the past 35 years, our community has grown many-fold – it's now too large to fit around my table or even within my home. But we still really need to encourage and help each other.

I hope this book encourages and supports you - and everyone you love - in Living with Addison's Disease.

Take care,

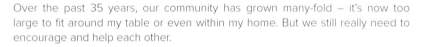

Deana Kenward MBE
Founder & Patron
Addison's Disease Self-Help Group
Guildford, United Kingdom
February 2019

Editor's Note

This book has been a ground-breaking project for people affected by Addison's disease.

We simply couldn't have taken it on without the goodwill, hard work and encouragement of lots of people in the Addison's community. We're indebted to many people, whose many years of advocacy and encouragement have made this book a joy to work on.

We're especially grateful to our core contributors, Professor Simon Pearce and Sarah Spain. They have worked tirelessly to combine medical accuracy with those essential and practical day-to-day aspects of living well with Addison's.

We are grateful to our medical contributors and clinical advisers, including Professor John Wass, Dr Vicki Rouse, Phillip Yeoh and Dr Tim Cheetham. We rely so much on your expertise and passion for patient care – thank you.

A special mention also goes to all our charity's members, volunteers, trustees and the wider team of contributors, who have worked so hard to bring this book to fruition. We welcome your comments and feedback – drop us a line at **ideas@addisons.org.uk** and share your thoughts.

Thank you everyone – you can be justly proud of your efforts!

Neil McClements
Editor
London
United Kingdom
February 2019

Our Authors

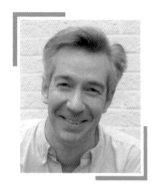

Simon Pearce is Professor of Endocrinology at Newcastle University (UK), affiliated to the Institute of Genetic Medicine and the Royal Victoria Infirmary (part of the Newcastle Hospitals NHS Foundation Trust), where he is an Honorary Consultant. He qualified in medicine from Newcastle University and undertook postgraduate training in endocrinology at the Royal Postgraduate Medical School, Hammersmith Hospital, London; Brigham & Women's Hospital, Boston, USA; and as a Wellcome Trust advanced research fellow in Newcastle. He published his first research paper on Addison's disease in 1998 and since then has been working to improve understanding of and treatment for the condition.

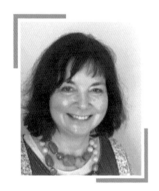

Sarah Spain MA MSc was diagnosed with Addison's Disease in her early 30s. A published author, she has an academic as well as a personal interest in the experience of long-term conditions and, particularly, issues surrounding health and social inequalities. For many years, she has contributed as a patient advocate and lay voice on several committees, for NICE (National Institute for Health and Care Excellence), the Royal College of Physicians, NHS England and OCDEM (Oxford Centre for Diabetes Endocrinology & Diabetes) based at Churchill Hospital, Oxford. She is co-founder of ELFy Apps, designed to support people who take daily medication.

Our Contributors

John Wass is a Professor of Endocrinology at Oxford University and was the Head of the Department of Endocrinology at the Oxford Centre for Diabetes, Endocrinology and Metabolism (OCDEM), Churchill Hospital Oxford, UK until 2011. From 1989 he was Professor of Clinical Endocrinology and Sub-Dean, University of London at Bart's. John Wass is currently the Clinical Reference Group Chair for Endocrinology in the UK.

Victoria Rouse is a GP working in Gateshead. She studied Medicine at Newcastle University, and did most of her postgraduate training in the North East. She was diagnosed with Type 1 diabetes as a child, and then diagnosed with Addison's disease during the first few years of working as a junior doctor. She later trained as a GP, and then worked in South Tyneside for 15 years, before relocating to Gateshead. She is interested in working in partnership with people with long term conditions to improve their care.

Tim Cheetham is Reader in Paediatric Endocrinology and Honorary Consultant Paediatrician at the Great North Children's Hospital in Newcastle. Tim's research activity reflects an interest in a range of clinical paediatric endocrine topics. His current roles include Chair of the congenital hypothyroidism advisory board, member of the BSPED studies group, associate editor of Archives of Disease in Childhood. He also answers patient / family queries submitted to the British Thyroid Foundation.

Phillip Yeoh is Consultant Nurse in Endocrinology at The London Clinic, a charity and independent hospital. Philip is Nurse Committee member for the Society for Endocrinology and a past Nurse Committee member at the European Society for Endocrinology. He has embarked on a PhD doctoral research programme in Health Studies/Nursing, specialising in the self-management of endocrine cancers.

Neil McClements joined the Addison's Disease Self-Help Group in October 2018 as Chief Executive. He is a board member of Haemochromatosis UK and a trustee of the British Liver Trust. In 2018, he was winner of the inaugural national Patient Safety Learning Awards and was a finalist in the AbbVie Better Health Awards. Neil is Patient Advisor to the NHS Primary Care Digital Transformation Clinical Advisory Group.

The Editor is grateful to **Hannah Kerr-Peterson** and **Lincoln Tsang** of **Arnold & Porter LLP** and the **Thomson Reuters Foundation** for their support with legal advice.

At A Glance Summary

▶ People with Addison's disease lack the adrenal hormones, cortisol and aldosterone, that are essential for life.

▶ Cortisol and aldosterone are usually replaced with hydrocortisone and fludrocortisone tablets, and you will have to take 2 or more doses of these every day for the rest of your life.

▶ It is important that you never run out of medication so make sure you have a secure supply at all times.

▶ Carry a steroid card and medical alert jewellery, in case you become confused or unconscious.

▶ If you become ill, you will need to increase the dose of your tablets for a day or two, or sometimes longer depending on the nature of the illness. Learn these 'sick-day rules' and stick to them.

▶ If you can't take the steroid tablets (eg. vomiting), you will need to have an injection instead.

▶ Make sure you, your family, friends or work colleagues know what to do if you need an injection.

▶ If you feel poorly, don't ignore it; take immediate action with extra medication. Be quick to seek help, if you need it.

▶ Addison's is a rare condition. Sometimes you will have to be your own medical expert as not all ambulance crew, nurses or doctors will be experienced with what to do.

▶ If you have a crisis and there is any doubt about the right management, insist on hydrocortisone 100mg by injection every 6 to 8 hrs and a saline drip, as this will always keep you safe.

▶ With the right medication, most people with Addison's lead close to normal lives. You can hold down a demanding job, have a family, travel the world or be a high-performing sports-person.

ADRENAL CRISIS CAN KILL

Read & understand the signs of Adrenal Crisis in Appendix E and the Sick Day Rules in Appendix F at the end of this book

Get educated, stay informed & keep safe.

Further Information & Resources

The Addison's Disease Self-Help Group (ADSHG) publishes a wide range of resources, for free download, from www.addisonsdisease.org.uk. These include :

- ▶ Diagnosing Addison's : A Guide For GPs

- ▶ Caring For Patients With Addison's : A Guide For GPs

- ▶ Managing Your Addison's : A Guide For People With Addison's Disease

- ▶ When A Student Has Addison's : A Guide For Schools & Parents

- ▶ ADSHG Surgical Guidelines (for people planning surgery, dentistry or other procedures)

- ▶ Nursing The Addison's Patient : Notes for Nurses

- ▶ When An Employee Has Addison's : A Guide For Employers

Join the Addison's Disease Self-Help Group

The Addison's Disease Self-Help Group is a UK registered charity and relies upon public subscriptions to support its work.

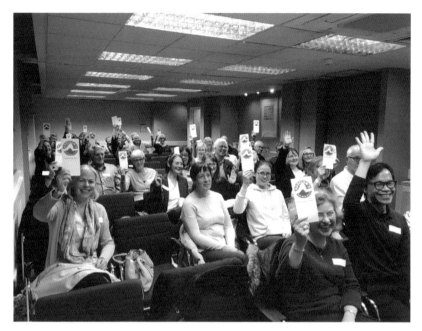

Some of our members, Glasgow, November 2018.

Membership is available globally for anyone affected by Addison's Disease, including patients, carers and clinicians. Membership provides a range of additional publications, support and services including online, private forums for mutual self-help and discussion of issues raised in this book.

To join us, go to **www.addisonsdisease.org.uk** .

Together, we are stronger.

1

Managing Your Addison's: An Introduction

Addison's is a rare endocrine condition where the adrenal glands cease to function, so that your body no longer produces enough of certain essential hormones, known as steroid hormones.

Fortunately, you can replace these essential hormones with daily steroid tablets. The hormones that your body no longer produces enough of are:

▶ Cortisol, aldosterone and DHEA (for "primary adrenal insufficiency" or Addison's disease)

▶ Cortisol and DHEA (in the case of "secondary adrenal insufficiency")

Cortisol regulates appetite, blood sugar and food metabolism; aldosterone regulates sodium, fluid balance and blood pressure; DHEA influences body hair growth and libido (sex drive). With the right balance of daily medication, people with Addison's can expect to have a normal life span and to lead full and productive lives. It is not unknown for people with Addison's to live into their 90s. Perhaps the most famous person with Addison's was US President John F Kennedy.

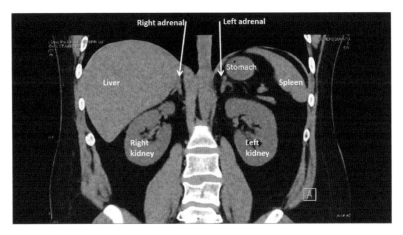

Addison's disease is caused when the adrenal glands no longer function correctly.

It takes time to adjust to a diagnosis of a long-term condition and you may not have heard of Addison's disease, prior to being diagnosed. Sometimes, owing to the non-specific nature of the symptoms (such as tiredness, dizziness, weight loss), the path to diagnosis is not straightforward. One study found that people with symptoms of Addison's disease had seen an average of 3 different doctors before the correct diagnosis was made.[1] After the diagnosis there can be a sense of relief, as well as uncertainty about what to expect in terms of living with the condition.

This guide has been written to help you manage your condition day-to-day. It provides information on what to do when you experience illness or other situations requiring extra care or short-term adjustments in medication. We hope that it will help reassure and inform you on this journey, especially when you are newly diagnosed. We trust that it will also serve as a useful reference for you and your family members over the longer term.

Because Addison's disease is rare, not all healthcare providers will have heard of it, and few will have a lot of experience. This means that it is important for you to know as much as possible, yourself. Nevertheless, this publication can only give you general advice and it cannot be a substitute for your own medical team assessing your individual healthcare needs.

Why is it called Addison's disease?

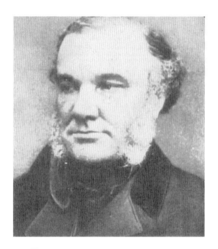

Dr Thomas Addison, 1793-1860

The condition is named after Thomas Addison, the London doctor who first identified the condition around 1850. Among people of European descent, it affects around 140 people per million. In the UK, that means around 9,000 people have been diagnosed with the condition. Although it is classified as a disease, it is neither infectious, nor easily inherited. In modern medical terminology, the condition is often described as primary adrenal insufficiency. Secondary adrenal insufficiency gives similar problems to Addison's disease

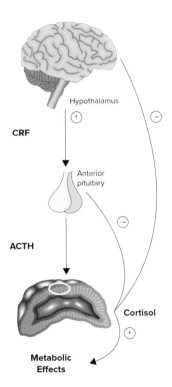

The pituitary gland controls what your adrenal glands do.

in that the adrenal glands fail to make cortisol and DHEA. However, secondary adrenal insufficiency is usually due to problems with the pituitary gland, which sits an inch behind the bridge of your nose, at the base of the brain. The pituitary gland makes a substance called ACTH (adrenocorticotropic hormone) which controls what your adrenal glands do. Anything that interrupts the ACTH supply to your adrenals can cause secondary adrenal insufficiency.

How is Addison's diagnosed?

Diagnosis is done by hospital blood tests and an assessment of your symptoms. The main blood test measures how much (or how little) cortisol your body can produce. It is called a Synacthen (ACTH stimulation) test.

Additional hospital blood tests will measure your aldosterone function. These are plasma renin, sodium & potassium tests. A further antibody blood test to establish the cause of your adrenal failure is recommended. If this is negative, an adrenal scan and other tests may be needed.

What causes Addison's disease?

In the developed world, 90% of people with primary adrenal insufficiency are suffering from an autoimmune condition. This is autoimmune Addison's disease and the body's immune system attacks and destroys both your adrenal glands over many months, leading to deficiency of the hormones. The adrenal antibody blood test can confirm that this is the cause of your problem.

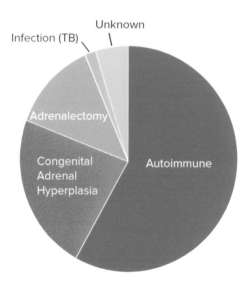

Causes of primary adrenal failure in the UK.

The second commonest cause is infections, particularly tuberculosis, some fungi and HIV-related infections: these bugs destroy the adrenal tissue too. Rarely, some tumours can squash both the adrenal glands, also leading to adrenal failure. If your blood antibody test is negative, you should have an adrenal scan to look for infections or tumours.

There are also a few people who are born with genetic problems in the steroid production equipment in their adrenal glands: the most common version of this is called congenital adrenal hyperplasia (CAH). However, many different, rare genetic diseases are known about, including adrenoleukodystrophy (ALD), which mainly affects boys and is associated with a deterioration in movement and brain functioning. These genetic conditions usually come to light in childhood.

Secondary adrenal insufficiency owing to ACTH deficiency is about 4 times more prevalent than primary Addison's disease and pituitary tumours are the commonest cause. Adrenal suppression due to taking steroid tablets is also very common (sometimes called "tertiary adrenal insufficiency").

Type of adrenal failure	What has gone wrong?	Missing adrenal hormones
Primary	Adrenal glands directly destroyed/ malfunction	Cortisol, Aldosterone, DHEA
Secondary	Pituitary problem giving deficient ACTH production	Cortisol, DHEA
Tertiary	Steroid medication use leading to low ACTH	Cortisol, DHEA

2

You and Your Doctors

You and your endocrinology team

Your endocrinology team has primary responsibility for monitoring your Addison's, including reviewing your medication needs, checking for any changes in your condition and also for any signs of other, related autoimmune conditions, such as diabetes or thyroid problems.

Generally speaking, you should expect to have this kind of review once or twice a year. After each consultation, your endocrinologist will write to you and your general practitioner (GP) with a summary of the consultation, the results of any blood tests you may have had and, if appropriate, any further recommended action.

Because you have to take steroid medications every day of your life, you will need to carry a steroid card, which identifies to healthcare providers that your medication cannot be stopped. It is also recommended to carry some medical identification jewellery, such a bracelet, necklace or dog-tag, that has information about your diagnosis and medication needs. These are important as if you become seriously ill or unconscious, you may not be able to communicate your health problems effectively.

You should expect to be issued with an emergency kit by your endocrinology team, soon after you are diagnosed and are still under specialist care. This consists of an ampoule of hydrocortisone with a needle and syringe. You will also be guided on 'sick-day rules' and shown how to administer an emergency injection, should this become necessary. More details on all of this can be found in Appendix F.

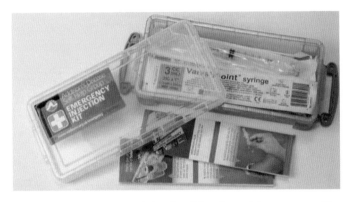

Always carry an emergency injection kit – it could save your life.

The Addison's Disease Self-Help Group (ADSHG) website has injection videos, diagrams and resources for you to view at **www.addisonsdisease.org.uk**. It is important that you familiarise yourself with your injection kit. It's also helpful if your partner, family members and work colleagues are also familiar with your emergency kit and how to use it. If you need someone to go over the injections with you or your family, the endocrine nurse in your endocrine centre (or the practice nurse at your local GP surgery) should be able to help.

You and your GP

On a day-to-day basis and for minor health issues not necessarily related to Addison's, your GP remains your main point of contact.

Not all GPs will be familiar with Addison's disease and the creation of a good working dialogue between you, your GP and your endocrinology team is really worthwhile. It will help particularly in situations where an unrelated illness may affect your Addison's. The Addison's Disease Self-Help Group (ADSHG) website has a range of publications and resources for GPs, including an introduction to Addison's Disease and "Caring for the patient with Addison's : a guide for GPs". These are available for free download at **www.addisonsdisease.org.uk**

Your GP is responsible for routinely prescribing your steroid replacement medicine – usually hydrocortisone and fludrocortisone – in the form of tablets. The *minimum* prescription recommended in the NHS England service specification for specialised endocrinology is 56 days. However, a repeat prescription length of 6 months at a time is preferable for essential steroid medications, in case of unexpected supply shortages. You must make sure that you never run out of medication, so try and keep a small stockpile with at least a month in reserve.

If you find that your GP is unwilling to issue a prescription for longer than 28 days (owing to guidelines set by their local Clinical Commissioning Group (CCG)), you could ask your endocrinologist to write and explain the reasons for a longer prescription. Alternatively, you could show your GP the Addison's Disease Self-Help Group letter written to the British Medical Journal (BMJ) explaining that an adequate supply of medication at all times is essential. The letter may be downloaded from www.addisonsdisease.org.uk. The Addison's Disease Self-Help Group is continuing to campaign to raise awareness and understanding of this issue, both at Government and CCG levels.

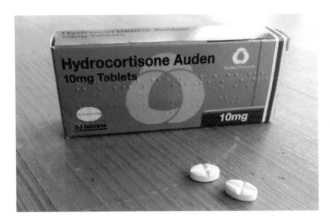

Hydrocortisone tablets.

Your GP will also subsequently prescribe replacement emergency ampoules, when they reach their expiry date, or if they have been used. It is important that you make a note of the expiry date, ideally when you pick up your medication. Your GP will also prescribe anti-nausea tablets or suppositories, as part of your emergency kit. While less critical, it is worth making a note of the expiry date on these too.

Replacement intramuscular needles are not available on prescription, but practice nurses typically have a supply to hand and will usually be willing to provide you with some of these on request. You may also be able to get a small number from your endocrine nurse, when you have your review, for instance.

However, you can also purchase intramuscular needles at cost from the Addison's Disease Self-Help Group shop (https://www.addisonsdisease.org.uk/shop), or from most pharmacies. Some Superdrug stores provide them for free, so it is worth asking.

For safety and convenience, you may want to request a small sharps bin from your GP. Sharps disposal is usually done by your local council, or you can hand the bin into a pharmacy, where they will empty it safely for you.

Exemption from prescription charges

Prescriptions are issued free of charge in Scotland, Wales and Northern Ireland.

In England, your GP can authorise a prescription exemption certificate for you. The application form is called 'FP92' and this is often kept in the practice or in pharmacies. Pick one up, fill in your details and get your GP to sign and stamp it. You will receive a reminder when your exemption certificate (in the form of a card) is nearing its expiry date, so that you can renew it in good time.

In the Republic of Ireland, patients with Addison's may be eligible for a Medical Card (means tested). Presently, Addison's disease is not covered under the Long Term Illness Scheme. See www.hse.ie

Ambulance trust registration

Your GP will also be able to help you register with your local ambulance trust. The information GPs pass on to the ambulance service is called a 'special patient note'. It is a good idea to contact your local ambulance service first to find out what is required, as this does vary from trust to trust – and not all GPs will be familiar with the process.

This measure should help ensure that you are either 'red-flagged' as a patient with Addison's, or that the first response vehicles in your area all carry injectable hydrocortisone and know how to use it.

You can find contact details of your local trust on the NHS Choices website for England (see https://www.nhs.uk/servicedirectories/pages/nhstrustlisting.aspx) and **www.ambulance.wales.nhs.uk** for Wales. For Scotland, this registration must be completed by your GP. Registration is not yet possible in Ireland, Northern Ireland or parts of Yorkshire.

Flu vaccine

You are strongly recommended to receive the annual winter flu vaccine. Flu-like infections cause about 10% of adrenal crises in people who are steroid-dependent. Within the UK, the annual winter flu vaccine is usually available, without charge, to people who are steroid-dependent. You may have to request this, rather than expect a routine reminder letter, and so it is a good idea to make a diary note for, say, late September, to contact your GP surgery.

In the Republic of Ireland, you must pay for this annual flu vaccine.

You and your dentist

Make sure that your dentist knows you have Addison's and that you will need extra cover, ranging from an extra hydrocortisone dose prior to minor procedures such as a replacement filling, to more significant extra cover for a tooth extraction, or during a course of antibiotics for a tooth abscess.

More details are provided in the ADSHG Surgical Guidelines leaflet available at **www.addisonsdisease.org.uk**.

3

Medication

What You Need And Why You Need It

Your adrenal glands make two hormones that are essential for life, called cortisol and aldosterone and these are steroid hormones. The healthy adrenal glands make cortisol in a specific daily rhythm and your treatment will roughly mirror the natural pattern of hormones manufactured by the adrenals.

In health, the concentration of cortisol in the blood starts to rise about 03:00hrs, peaking between 06:30 and 08:00 in most people. This surge of cortisol in the morning is what wakes most people from sleep. Cortisol production tails off after lunchtime, and by the late evening people have much lower levels and this makes you want to go back to sleep.

Each day most people with Addison's disease need to take a combination of **hydrocortisone** and **fludrocortisone** tablets to replace the missing cortisol and aldosterone hormones. While there are a few alternatives to hydrocortisone tablets, the only medication that replaces aldosterone is fludrocortisone. People can need quite different doses of these steroid tablets, and this depends on body size, age and level of activity. Your endocrinologist will have a reasonable idea of a good starting dose for you, and then your medication can be fine-tuned over a few weeks or months to get you feeling as good as possible. This

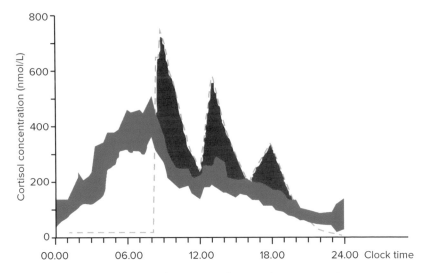

The blue area represents the range of cortisol concentrations over the course of a day in healthy people. The red areas is the estimated cortisol levels in people taking 3 doses of hydrocortisone daily.

might involve taking your medication at slightly different times of day, as well as changing the dose.

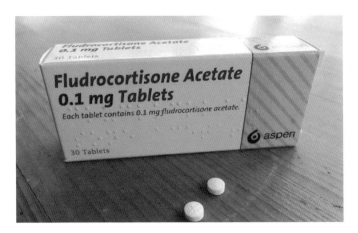

Fludrocortisone tablets.

Even once you are established on a regimen of medication that suits you, it is possible for this to change over time. You will need to be seen regularly (normally once or twice each year) by your endocrinology team to keep an eye on how you feel.

Cortisol Replacement

People who are cortisol deficient feel exhausted, often with nausea, no appetite, vomiting and weight loss. **Hydrocortisone** is the chemical name for cortisol once it has been made into a drug-it is exactly the same as natural cortisol. Hydrocortisone tablets are usually taken twice or three times daily. In general, a 'little and often' dose works best and gives a steadier level of cortisol in your blood. The first dose of hydrocortisone is usually the biggest and should be taken immediately when you wake up and preferably before you get out of bed. Subsequent doses are usually smaller.

It takes 20 to 30 minutes to start to absorb a hydrocortisone tablet from your stomach and the speed isn't greatly affected by whether you have eaten or not. Doses of 20mgs or less do not have to be taken with food, unless you have trouble digesting these. A single hydrocortisone dose will produce adequate hormone levels for 4 to 6 hours in most people, meaning your next dose should be 4 to 6 hours later. You are advised to take the last dose of hydrocortisone four to six hours before bedtime, as taking it later leads to higher than normal evening levels and may keep you awake. Many people use mobile phone alarms to remind them to take their doses each day.

The main theoretical advantage of the alternative medications to hydrocortisone is that they last for longer in your body. Hydrocortisone is the natural hormone, and your body gets rid of it quite quickly. In contrast taking **prednisolone** or **dexamethasone**, which are the alternatives and last for much longer, means you may be able to take just one dose each day. As well as replacing cortisol, hydrocortisone has some hormonal action that overlaps with that of aldosterone. This means that if you switch from hydrocortisone to dexamethasone, you will need to increase your dose of fludrocortisone. This is also possible in a swap from hydrocortisone to prednisolone, but the effect is less marked.

Although steroid medication is life-saving and life-sustaining for someone with Addison's disease, if taken in too high a dose or at the wrong time of day, it can lead to side effects or complications over many years.

There are two main reasons that most endocrinologists feel more comfortable prescribing hydrocortisone than the alternatives. Firstly, the short half-life in your body means it doesn't accumulate and is the body's natural product. Secondly, there are more than fifty years of experience using hydrocortisone in adrenally

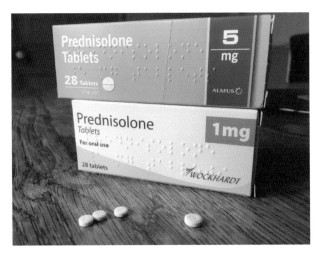

Prednisolone tablets.

insufficient patients, giving the most confidence about the risk of long-term complications during the course of a lifetime.

A fourth medication that can be used for cortisol replacement is called **cortisone acetate**. This was the original adrenal steroid discovered during the 1940s and has been largely superseded by hydrocortisone except in a few countries. Cortisone acetate can be considered a precursor drug for hydrocortisone, as it needs to be activated by the liver and other tissues for it to become active.

Each of these other drugs has a different strength (officially called 'potency') compared to hydrocortisone; roughly equivalent doses are shown in the table below.[2]

Equivalent doses of different cortisol replacement tablets

Drug	Equivalent dose	Split into daily doses
Hydrocortisone	20mg	2 or 3 doses
Prednisolone	5mg	1 (or 2)
Dexamethasone*	0.75mg	1 or 2
Cortisone acetate	25mg	2 or 3

*Although dexamethasone is a theoretical replacement steroid, its long duration of action and the high denomination of tablet strengths means most people who take it end up overdosed, and so it isn't recommended in most circumstances.

What Are The Considerations In Choosing Cortisol Replacement?

Essentially, in the UK your choice is between **hydrocortisone** and **prednisolone**. If you feel well while taking 2 or 3 doses of hydrocortisone daily, this is probably the safest treatment to stick with in the long term. On the other hand, if you have fluctuations in energy during the day that stop you doing what you would like, or you have a job where taking a lunchtime dose of medication is virtually impossible, then you may consider prednisolone.[3] Prednisolone might also be suitable for young adults, where both the practicalities of taking a lunchtime dose in school hours, and the social discomfort that some younger people feel around illness may make a once daily prednisolone dose an attractive option. If you don't feel perfect on hydrocortisone then you should consider trying the alternative and see if it improves things for you, but think of it as a non-binding trial of the medication. If it doesn't work for you after a 7 day trial, go back on your original regimen.

Example hydrocortisone dose regimens.

Name	Job	Weight	Work hours	Hydrocortisone doses (Time, dose)			
Lois	Journalist	49kg	9-5	07:30, 10mg	12:00, 5mg	-	-
Darlene	Student	52kg	8-5	07:00, 7.5mg	12:00, 5mg	16:00, 2.5mg	*
Jackie	Nurse	59kg	8-8	07:00, 10mg	11:00, 2.5mg	14:00, 2.5mg	18:00, 2.5mg
Patrick	Postman	65kg	6-3	05:00, 10mg	10:00, 5mg	15:00, 2.5mg	-
Lynette	Housewife	76kg	7-7	06:30, 10mg	12:00, 10mg	†	-
Steve	IT tech	78kg	9-5	07:30, 10mg	13:00, 5mg	16:00, 5mg	§
David	Night porter	85kg	10pm-6	20:00, 10mg	01:00, 5mg	05:00, 5mg	-
Robert	Builder	104kg	8-4	06:00, 10mg	11:00, 10mg	16:00, 5mg	-

*Darlene goes to a 60 min spin class on 2 evenings each week and takes an extra 2.5mg at the start. She goes dancing with friends on Friday nights and takes an extra 5mg at 20:00hrs.

†Lynette goes to Pilates on Wednesday afternoon and splits her 10mg 12:00 dose to 5mg+5mg so she can take some just before the class

§Steve has to stay late during certain work projects and takes an extra 5mg at 19:00 if he has to work until 21:00

Having a relatively fixed routine in your daily hydrocortisone schedule will allow you to fine-tune the doses to get you feeling predictably well each day. However, as no one does the same thing on seven days a week, a degree of flexibility may be needed to accommodate small changes in what you do each day.

On a weekend, many people will take their morning dose of hydrocortisone an hour or two later and knock on the rest of their day's doses. Similarly, if you do some exercise after work or have to work longer hours, then you may find that you feel better splitting a dose or taking an extra dose later on. With these small dose changes, there is no right or wrong thing to do. However, you may be surprised that you can get away without changing your dose schedule for a wide variety of activities.

Remember that it is normal to feel tired after 8 hours at work or an hour in the gym, so don't expect to never feel tired - this is normal for everyone. You will learn to recognise the difference between feeling appropriately tired and feeling poorly.

Cortisol Replacement: The Small Print

One additional reason to prefer hydrocortisone is if you have a problem with tablet absorption from your stomach or guts. In fact, hydrocortisone is readily absorbed and even people with a significantly shortened bowel (eg. following surgery for weight loss) normally have no problem absorbing steroids.

Nevertheless, hydrocortisone is measurable in blood (as cortisol) and this can help guide your dosing if you have a significant gut absorption problem. A hydrocortisone 'day curve' can be performed in an endocrine ward, where you take your normal daily hydrocortisone tablets by mouth and you have blood taken 4 or 5 times during the day to measure the amount of cortisol absorbed into the blood. If the levels are too low, your doctor would use this to guide a dose increase.

For several years, drug companies have been developing different formulations of hydrocortisone to enable it to be taken as a once daily, slow-release tablet. Two such preparations are called **Plenadren**® and **Chronocort**®. Plenadren currently has an EU licence and is, in principle, available. However, in practice it is so expensive compared to regular hydrocortisone (about £300 per month) that it has been effectively banned by most local CCGs (Clinical Commissioning Groups). You may be able to obtain it if you are willing to pay for a private prescription or if you have special issues and your endocrinologist has a special local arrangement. Chronocort® has yet to receive a licence to be marketed in the UK. Hopefully NHS rules on these medications will relax in the future.

Recently, some centres have offered continuous subcutaneous hydrocortisone infusion (CSHI) where hydrocortisone solution is given via a pump into the subcutaneous (fat) tissue on your abdomen.

This method of hydrocortisone administration is an off-licence use but a big centre in Norway has been using this for over 10 years.[4] However, the published data remain patchy and the NHS is not funding this except for in very exceptional circumstances at the moment.

In this method of hydrocortisone delivery, hydrocortisone is given slowly throughout a 24 hour period, fluctuating according to the normal daily pattern. One of the risks of CSHI is infusion site infection. CSHI patients need to be aware of this risk and need to check the infusion site regularly, choosing a different infusion site and ensuring the right skin cleansing wipe is used to reduce this risk.

For young children and small babies with adrenal insufficiency, a granular preparation of hydrocortisone is available in sachets called **Alkindi**®. This allows young children and small babies to get an appropriate replacement steroid dose.

Aldosterone Replacement

People with Addison's disease (primary adrenal insufficiency) leak salt from their kidneys because of aldosterone deficiency. This leads to salt depletion, which results in low blood pressure, light-headedness, thirst, passing urine at night, back and muscle cramps, and salt craving.

Aldosterone is replaced with fludrocortisone tablets, which are usually taken as a single daily dose. As your body has several days' reserve of salt, it can feel like the fludrocortisone tablet doesn't do very much, as if you miss one or two doses you won't feel immediately ill. In addition, some people can partially compensate for fludrocortisone under-dosing by increasing their salt intake. However, it is important to take your fludrocortisone as prescribed, as salt-depletion can make you feel chronically washed-out and exhausted.

People with Addison's disease and other causes of primary adrenal insufficiency should take as much salt as they feel like eating: the usual healthy eating restriction on salt intake doesn't apply. In addition to salt craving, people with aldosterone deficiency sometimes have characteristic taste preferences for pickled foods, vinegar and sour foods, such as lemons or Granny Smith apples.

The average dose of fludrocortisone is 100mcg daily (100 micrograms, also written as 0.1 milligrams [mg]), which is one tablet daily for most people. Younger people and people who are physically active characteristically need more and doses of up to 600mcg daily are occasionally necessary. In contrast, older people may often feel well just taking half a tablet (50mcg) daily.

Most people take their fludrocortisone on waking with their first dose of hydrocortisone, but because of the long duration of the effects, it can be taken at any time of day. In addition, a few children and younger people need to take salt tablets (sodium chloride) each day to keep well.

If you travel to a hot environment where you are sweating more, your body will lose more salt. In this situation, local foods are often saltier, but you may also need to increase your fludrocortisone dose and keep up your salt intake. A reliable sign that you need to take more fludrocortisone is if you start to feel light-headed; this is usually preceded by a feeling of being washed out and drained. In contrast, people who have taken too much fludrocortisone and/ or salt get foot and ankle swelling, and this is not uncommon after a period of hospital treatment with a saline drip for their Addison's disease. People with Addison's disease also need to avoid taking licorice, as this has an effect like fludrocortisone and the combination can make your ankles and legs swell up.

A small number of people with adrenal insufficiency do not need to take fludrocortisone once their hydrocortisone medication is stable. However, this is unusual in autoimmune Addison's disease and suggests a different cause for adrenal insufficiency.

People with secondary adrenal failure, which is due to pituitary disease, do not usually need to take fludrocortisone. Similarly, individuals who are experiencing steroid medication-induced adrenal suppression do not need to take fludrocortisone.

Monitoring

People with adrenal insufficiency should be seen regularly by the endocrinology team in the first few months after the diagnosis to make sure they are feeling well and are confident about what to do with their medication in the event of an illness or emergency (see 'sick-day rules' in Appendix F).

After this initial period, it is normally satisfactory to have a once or twice yearly review appointment. This review appointment is your chance to let the doctor know how you are feeling, what is going well, and what you can't do but would like to be able to.

Be honest with your doctor about your tablets; everyone misses the occasional medication dose and doctors won't be surprised by this. If you find out by accident that you can miss out your 16:00 hydrocortisone dose and still feel fine during the evening and the next morning, this is important information to tell your doctor. Similarly, if you feel rubbish at 11:30 most days and your next hydrocortisone dose isn't due until 13:00, let your doctor know. The information is hugely valuable in fine-tuning your doses so you feel the best possible. You might find it helpful to make a short 'reminder' list of your main concerns or questions, ahead of your review. Don't worry if some of these seem trivial. They can often be helpful clues and so are worth mentioning.

During the appointment, you should have your weight taken and your blood pressure measured lying down and standing up. Low blood pressure, or a fall in blood pressure on standing, can mean too little fludrocortisone. Similarly, too much weight gain can indicate a reduction in hydrocortisone is warranted.

You should have a blood test for the blood salt levels and kidney function, which is called urea and electrolytes or U&E for short. If your blood sodium is low, this would indicate that more fludrocortisone is needed. A surrogate indicator of the amount of salt in your body is another blood test called renin, which really measures blood flow to your kidneys. A slightly high renin can be normal if you are dehydrated and thirsty, but it may also indicate that your fludrocortisone dose should be increased.

In addition to having a blood test once or twice yearly to check that your hydrocortisone and fludrocortisone doses are OK, your endocrinologist may like to check that you haven't developed any other conditions.

Some other autoimmune conditions are found quite commonly in people with Addison's disease and it makes sense to look for these occasionally. For instance, more than 50% of Addison's patients will have a thyroid problem, either before or after diagnosis, and it is reasonable to check your thyroid blood tests once a year. Occasionally in women the ovaries stop working and absent periods will develop. This can also be autoimmune (see fertility section).

Hypothyroidism (45%)

Graves' disease (15%)

Pernicious anaemia (20%)

Type 1 diabetes (10%)

Premature ovarian failure (10%)

Vitiligo (5%)

Coeliac disease (5%)

Other autoimmune conditions with Addison's disease.

Other autoimmune conditions may be predicted by measuring blood antibodies, such as type 1 diabetes or coeliac disease. The risks of these conditions vary depending on your age, gender and what else is wrong with you. In some situations, for instance in children and teenagers, it is a good idea to check for type 1 diabetes antibodies.

Other conditions, particularly osteoporosis and type 2 diabetes, may occur as a complication of being treated with steroid medications for a long time. Your doctor may arrange a bone (DEXA) scan to look for osteoporosis every 5 years, or check your blood for the average sugar levels (the glycosylated haemoglobin or HbA1c test).

Remember that although you might not have an appointment scheduled for another 12 months, if you start to feel poorly, it is reasonable to contact the endocrine team to get advice in the meantime. Often the endocrine specialist nurse may be able to help you, or accelerate your next appointment with the consultant. Don't be afraid to ask.

Drug Interactions

Most prescription and over the counter drugs do not affect your steroid medication, although it is always wise to check this with your doctor or pharmacist. However, there are a few prescription drugs that influence the way hydrocortisone and other steroid medications are handled by the body, either slowing down or speeding up the rate at which the steroids are metabolised. This means that people taking certain drugs may need to adjust their steroid medications.

Anti-epilepsy medications (typically carbamazepine, phenytoin and topiramate) speed up the metabolism of hydrocortisone, and some people need to take 30-50% higher doses during such treatment.

Occasionally adrenal insufficiency is caused by tuberculosis of the adrenal glands. Anyone who is taking rifampicin or rifabutin to treat tuberculosis may need to increase their dose of both hydrocortisone and fludrocortisone by up to double the normal dose. In a similar way to the epilepsy medications, these anti-tuberculosis drugs speed up the rate at which the body destroys the steroid medication. Growth hormone treatment can lower blood levels of cortisol and oestrogen, and oral contraceptive pills can increase the blood level of cortisol.

Some drugs that are used to treat HIV infection such as ritonavir can stop steroid excretion, leading to manifestations of severe steroid excess. In this case, your regular hydrocortisone replacement might cause weight gain, high blood pressure and a puffy face and neck- features called Cushing's syndrome that are due to build-up of too much steroid in your body. Some anti-fungal drugs (itraconazole) may have the same effect.

Replacement Of Other Adrenal Hormones?

As well as making cortisol and aldosterone, your adrenal glands also make a series of hormones called adrenal androgens or sex steroids. People with Addison's disease are deficient in these hormones too. The effect of this seems very minimal in men, as the testicles continue to produce androgens as normal. However, in women, particularly after the menopause, lack of adrenal androgens causes the underarm hair to stop growing and may also affect sex drive. The main component of the adrenal androgens is called dehydroepiandrosterone and even endocrinologists tend to abbreviate this to DHEA. Adrenal DHEA production is measured in the blood by measuring its derivative DHEAS (S stands for sulfate).

Several clinical trials replacing DHEA in people with adrenal insufficiency have been performed and there is not a clear-cut benefit for most people.[5] Nevertheless, occasionally women do clearly feel better on DHEA tablets and so it should not be discounted.

However, there are side effects and complications. Many people will see a more oily or greasy skin (this can be welcome if you start with dry skin), but acne and pimples can also develop. DHEA is also metabolised to oestrogen by the body, which may bring with it the risk of breast cancer, which has been found in a few women with Addison's disease taking DHEA. The ideal dose of DHEA is between 25 and 50mg in most women and this can be taken once

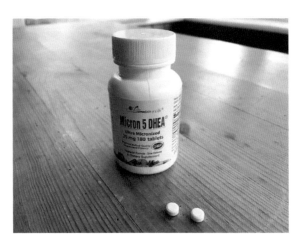

DHEA tablets.

daily. Some people may need a lower dose and a blood test to measure DHEAS is a simple way to judge this.

DHEA can't be prescribed on the NHS as it is classed as a food supplement. If you want to try it, discuss it with your doctor and then you will have to buy it from a pharmacy or health food store. Talk to your doctor or a pharmacist to find a reliable source of high quality DHEA, as the unregulated nature of these preparations means that not all are high quality.

Obtaining And Storing Medication

You need to obtain a good supply of your hydrocortisone and fludrocortisone tablets. Occasionally you will need to double your daily hydrocortisone doses according to 'sick-day rules' in Appendix F, so it is vital that you have at least a month's supply of tablets surplus to your basic daily requirement.

For this reason, it is recommended that you ask your GP to prescribe at least 56 days of medication and you should aim to keep a small stockpile. You must make sure that you never ever run out, as there have been tragic fatalities in people with Addison's who simply ran out of medication.

It used to be recommended to store some older formulations of fludrocortisone in the fridge: this wasn't really necessary (it just allowed the pharmacy to extend the 'expiry' date). Most current fludrocortisone tablets are stable at room temperature. Keep a few spare hydrocortisone tablets in your car, handbag, in your workplace and in your usual coat or jacket etc. This is essential for unexpected illness, as well as useful for when you are out and about.

Both your steroid tablets and hydrocortisone ampoules for injection will have an expiry date, which is like a 'use by' or 'best

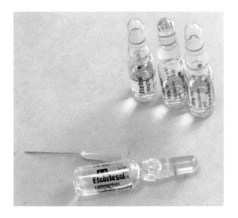

Hydrocortisone ampoules.

before' date on food. Keep a note of the expiry dates and replace the medicines with a fresh supply from your GP before the drug goes past this date.

In general, medications very slowly degrade even at the recommended storage temperature. This degradation is accelerated by humidity or heat. The expiry date refers to the longest time the pharmaceutical company has tested the tablets, powder or liquid formulation for stability. This means that a 100mg ampoule of hydrocortisone will likely still have 90mg of active hydrocortisone in it, even months after its expiry date. While it isn't ideal to have to use a medicine after its expiry date, you would still be much safer using an injection or tablets that are a few months past the expiry date than going without any medication.

Similarly, if you have to take medications to a hot environment and can't refrigerate them, keep them in the shade and as cool as possible. These medications will almost certainly work perfectly well for several weeks, but it would be sensible to replace them with a fresh supply when you get back home.

Adrenal Crisis & Emergencies

Each year, eight to ten percent of people with Addison's disease suffer an 'adrenal crisis', although around half of all people have never had an episode. Adrenal crisis is when the level of your steroid hormones becomes too low for your body's needs. You might feel terribly poorly, with low blood pressure, very fast or very slow heart rate, headache, vomiting, light-headedness, feeling very cold, confusion, drowsiness or loss of consciousness. **This is a medical emergency and you need to receive a hydrocortisone injection and a drip as soon as possible.**

When you are first diagnosed with adrenal insufficiency, your endocrinology team will provide you with a few ampoules of hydrocortisone (100mg), some needles and syringes.[*1] Injectable hydrocortisone comes either as a liquid, (called hydrocortisone sodium phosphate), or as a powder that has to be mixed with water before use (hydrocortisone succinate). Both work equally well, but the powder takes longer to prepare. Make a note of the expiry date of these ampoules, to ensure that they are replaced in good time. You will be taught how to inject yourself in the thigh or arm with hydrocortisone. Bring along your spouse, partner, friend or flat mate so that you have back up. Ask for refresher training at any stage if you aren't confident that you could do it. Nursing staff at some GP surgeries are able to undertake this for you, so you may not need to travel to a specialist centre. Several videos demonstrating how to give a hydrocortisone injection are available from the Addison's Disease Self-Help Group website www.addisonsdisease.org.uk .

---

[1] *If your endocrine team won't provide this for you, ask your GP for referral to a centre where the team has experience looking after people with Addison's disease.

Have you needed emergency treatement for adrenal crisis at any stage since your diagnosis? (hydrocortisone injection and/or IV fluids via a drip)

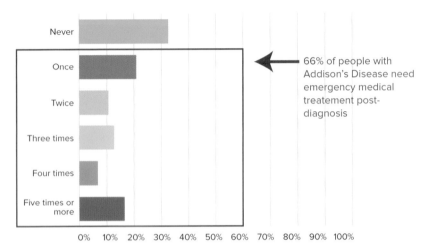

66% of people with Addison's Disease need emergency medical treatement post-diagnosis

Adrenal crisis is a critical medical emergency which the majority of people will experience at some stage.

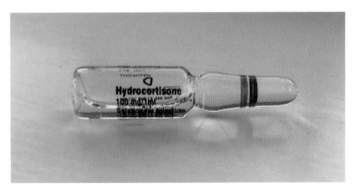

A hydrocortisone ampoule.

If you start to vomit and can't keep your tablets down, this is a potentially serious situation for someone with steroid medication dependency. You should try to take a double dose of your tablets again immediately and if you vomit them back within half an hour, you will need to have hydrocortisone by injection. The dose is the full 100mg ampoule for adults, but only half an ampoule (50mg) for primary school age children. There is a short video showing you how to do this on the ADSHG website and there is a leaflet available taking you through each of the steps as well.

After the injection, if you know why you are vomiting (eg. food poisoning, excess alcohol) then it may be OK just to ride it out for an hour or two to see if it settles down. However, if you feel light-headed, dizzy when you sit or stand, thirsty or drowsy then this indicates dehydration and if you can't keep liquids down, you will need to go to hospital for a saline drip as well.

If you sustain a significant injury, or start to feel really ill for any other reason, then you should also inject yourself with the hydrocortisone ampoule – or get someone else to do this for you. Light-headedness, fainting, drowsiness, feeling very cold or just plain 'terrible' all indicate adrenal crisis and that you need to have an immediate injection. **Inject yourself and then ring 999 (or 112/ 911)**; inform the call handler that you are having an **ADDISONIAN CRISIS** and to dispatch a team with hydrocortisone. Even if there is a delay in getting an ambulance to you, the injection means that you will be safe from the adrenal point of view for a few hours.

Bear in mind that Addison's disease is rare and that not all ambulance teams will be confident in managing your steroid needs. You (and/or a partner, spouse or friend) need to be prepared to stay 'in charge' of your own steroid-dependent situation, until you are comfortable that the medical team understand your needs.

Experience shows that there can be significant delays in giving hydrocortisone injections in busy hospital A&E departments, so

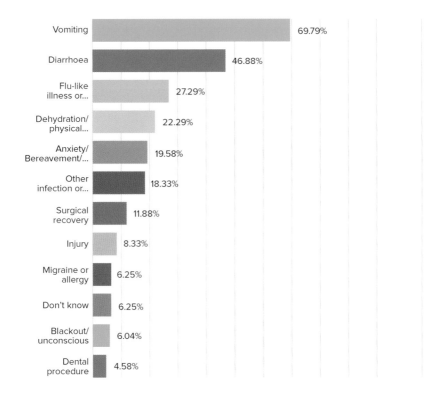

ADSHG Patient Survey 2018 (n=480)

Many things can trigger an adrenal crisis. A simple stomach bug can become a medical emergency, without proper care.

make yourself safe by giving your own (or having a partner, spouse or friend administer it) before you get hospital.[6]

Paradoxically, it can be a lot more difficult to self-medicate once you are in a hospital, even when you know that it is the right thing. If you possibly can, try and make sure you have a partner, spouse or friend accompanying you to hospital, so they can help communicate your steroid needs.

If you need significant dental work, minor medical procedures (eg. endoscopy, biopsy) or major surgery (with general anaesthesia), then you will need one or more injections. All the time that you are unable to take your steroid tablets by mouth during an illness or following an operation, you will need to have 3 injections of hydrocortisone daily. The alternative to this is a continuous intravenous infusion of hydrocortisone, 200mg over 24hrs. Make sure you discuss this with your dentist, surgeon and anaesthetist and give them a printout of the ADSHG surgical guidelines available at www.addisonsdisease.org.uk. Don't sign the consent form for the procedure until you are happy that the team understand your steroid-dependency.

Sick-Day Rules

When your body is stressed, either through a physical illness or injury, or due to a mental stress, a healthy person's adrenal glands will make more cortisol. This response is an important part of your body's natural mechanism to combat any illness or injury. When you have adrenal insufficiency, your body can't respond in the normal way, so you will need to take more hydrocortisone. In the best case, these extra 'stress' doses keep you feeling well during the illness or injury.

Failure to increase your hydrocortisone dose during a more severe illness or injury can lead to adrenal crisis. In several situations you will need to change your hydrocortisone dose.

You should double your daily hydrocortisone dose if:

▶ You get an infection with a temperature of 38.0°C or higher

▶ You get a bad cold, flu, diarrhoea or other infection that makes you feel poorly or weak

> ▶ You break a bone or suffer from any similar significant injury

Keep your dose of steroids doubled for 2 days and then go back to your usual dose. For example: if you take hydrocortisone 10mg on waking, 5mg at midday and 5mg in the evening increase these with an immediate dose of 20mg, followed by 10mg every six hours for 2 days or until you are feeling better.

If you take less than 20mg in total as your regular daily dose, go up to 40 or 50mg daily. Take a doubled dose when you first feel ill, or a minimum of 20mg. Follow this by doubling your doses for the rest of the day, or a minimum of 10mg continuing every 6 hours during stress and illness.

If you don't feel better after 48hrs, keep your hydrocortisone doubled and seek advice from your GP or your endocrine nurse or doctor. If you are prescribed antibiotics for an infection, double your hydrocortisone dose *until you finish the course.*

As well as physical illness or injury, severe psychological stress, such as attending the funeral of a loved one, may also require an increase in hydrocortisone dose.

If you get a severe infection with a temperature above 40.0°C, then you need to take 3 times your normal hydrocortisone dose and seek advice from your doctor immediately. This could be the start of an adrenal crisis.

When your hydrocortisone is doubled or trebled, the hydrocortisone has enough of an effect that you don't need to increase your fludrocortisone. However, if you feel light-headed or drained, topping up on your salt or eating soup may help you feel better.

Emergency Prevention

Vomiting and diarrhoea account for more than half of all adrenal crisis and emergency hospital admissions for patients with Addison's disease, so try to take sensible precautions to avoid these. Keep away from friends or relatives who have had a winter vomiting bug or stomach virus. Eat cautiously from street food vendors or the summer barbecue, and bear in mind that undercooked chicken is a lot more likely to harbour food-poisoning bugs than a steak or a veggie burger.

Suffering from any infection could precipitate an adrenal crisis. Many are unavoidable, but you can protect yourself from flu to some extent by getting your flu jab each September or October.

The other preventable cause of adrenal crises is that resulting from medical, dental and surgical interventions. Ask your surgeon/dentist/endoscopist to talk to your endocrinologist for advice ahead of any planned procedure. Whenever you can't take tablets ("nil-by-mouth"), you need to ensure that you get an injection of hydrocortisone at least every 8 hours. In addition, if you are having a significant procedure, you should have a hydrocortisone injection at the start of the anaesthetic. This applies to all procedures done under general anaesthetic and many that are done under local anaesthesia. Refer to the surgical guidelines and make sure your medical team have seen these. The Addison's Disease Self-Help Group publish detailed surgical guidelines for free download from **www.addisonsdisease.org.uk.**

If you have doubts about the provision of steroid cover for your procedure, ask to talk to the anaesthetist directly, involve your endocrinologist/endocrine nurse, and don't sign the consent form until you are satisfied it will be safe.

Keep good supplies of medication in your house, outdoor garments, handbag, sports bag and car, so that you are never stranded without. Be proactive in taking an extra dose of hydrocortisone (typically 5 or 10mg is enough) if you start to feel under the weather or poorly.

Make sure your friends, family or work colleagues alert you quickly if you start to look peaky or off-colour; after some experience, most will develop a good instinct for how you are feeling. Make sure the first-aiders in your work place know about your steroid-dependency and what to do if you need an emergency injection.

Plan your travels carefully and take enough extra tablet medication for the worst-case scenario, as well as your emergency injection kit.

Travelling (Both Near And Far)

Make sure that you have plenty of medication with you for the length of your travels and take extra, to cover the possibility that you might need to unexpectedly double the dose while you are away.

People do lose bags and coats while they are travelling, so keep a supply of tablets in your pocket or hand luggage, as well as in your cabin bag or suitcase if you are flying. Remember that you have to 'fail-safe', so consider plans such as giving a back-up supply to a travelling companion as well.

Don't forget to take your emergency hydrocortisone injection kit with you, too. Your endocrinologist or GP will provide a letter to confirm that you need to travel with syringes and needles, which will be needed at some customs and security checkpoints.

If you find yourself somewhere without medication, you will need to obtain a supply as quickly as possible. In the UK, a pharmacist will be able to ring your local pharmacy or your GP practice to confirm that you need the medication. Larger pharmacies also sell 2.5mg hydrocortisone lozenges which are called "Corlan" that are used to treat mouth ulcers without prescription ('over the counter'). You can make up your hydrocortisone dose with 2 or 4 Corlan and it works just as well when swallowed.

In many other countries, you can simply go into a pharmacy and buy hydrocortisone or prednisolone without a prescription. Bear in mind that the tablets could have a slightly different name or brand overseas, which might add to a communication barrier (eg. hidrocortizon or hidrocortisona etc.). In this situation, something is infinitely better than nothing, and prednisolone will definitely keep you alive, even if your normal medication is hydrocortisone and vice-versa. If you need a prescription to obtain steroid medications, then you will need to go to a hospital emergency department or seek an appointment with a local doctor. Show your steroid card and emergency identification tag/bracelet to make it obvious what you need.

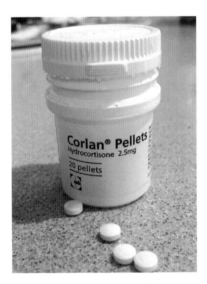

Corlan pellets are available over-the-counter from pharmacies

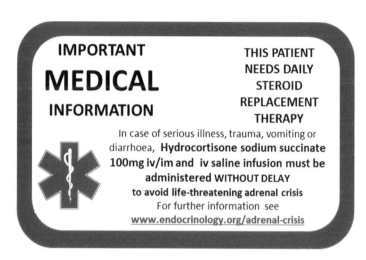

An EU steroid emergency card.

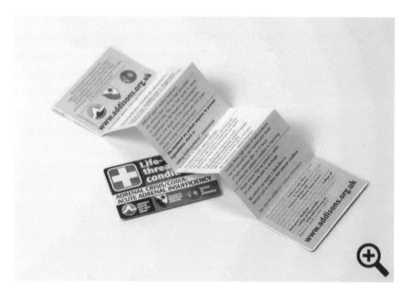

The ADSHG emergency card

4

What Kind of Quality of Life Can I Expect?

People with Addison's can expect to have a normal lifespan and, with careful management, a good quality of life (unless they have other medical complications). It is not unknown for people with Addison's to live into their 90s. With the right balance of medication and a reasonably healthy lifestyle, most people can more or less continue as normal, prior to diagnosis.

There are no restrictions on activities such as driving. It is a good idea to keep a second injection kit in the car, in case of injury. Within both the UK and the Republic of Ireland, you are only required to inform the licensing authority about your condition if you hold an HGV (group 2) licence. Where you have additional medical conditions, please check whether these must be declared.

Your private car insurance company may wish to be informed about your condition. You may well have to inform your travel insurance company, but this should not make you ineligible for cover. You can register as an organ donor, but it is not advisable to give blood. The fluid loss could be destabilising to your fludrocortisone (mineralocorticoid) dependency.

There is no need to adopt a special diet or any dietary restrictions, although a low-salt diet is best avoided. Grapefruit and real licorice can amplify the effects of your steroid medication and are not recommended.

However, it is true that most people – including those with exceptional fitness – do experience occasional episodes of unusual fatigue. At these times you will need to allow your body to catch up, with extra rest. Occasionally, if you become particularly tired (such as needing bedrest during the day) you may benefit from taking a small extra dose (around one-quarter of your daily dose should be sufficient), but be aware that too much extra steroid is not a good idea in the long term. Bear in mind that such an episode could also represent salt depletion, and having salty foods or something like soup to eat is a good way to combat this.

If you find you are experiencing these episodes on a regular basis, it would be reasonable to check this with your endocrinologist,

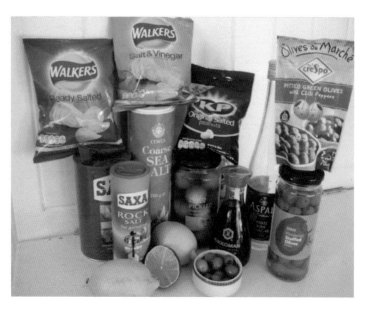

Craving salty, acidic and sour foods is common in people with Addison's.

to ensure that your medication regimen (timing and dosage) is the right one for you. Sometimes a modest adjustment to either the hydrocortisone or fludrocortisone can make a significant difference.

You can find more information on signs of being over- and under-medicated on page 51.

Fertility

Most women with Addison's can conceive normally.

However, in around 10% a problem with your ovaries can develop. The steroid hormones made by your adrenal glands share some similarities with oestrogens, which are also steroid hormones. This leads to cessation of menstrual periods in a small proportion of women with Addison's, a condition known as premature ovarian insufficiency. If this happens to you, it will cause problems with fertility.

Most men with Addison's don't have a problem conceiving.

Pregnancy

Most women need minimal changes in their steroid medications during pregnancy and with the right medical support, you can expect to have a healthy pregnancy and normal childbirth.[7] You should see your endocrinologist 3 or 4 times during the pregnancy to check things are going OK.

Early on in the pregnancy, morning sickness can stop you keeping the tablets down, and in severe cases you may need to inject yourself with hydrocortisone each morning for a week or two.

You also need particular attention paid to your blood pressure and blood sodium levels towards the end of pregnancy. The progesterone made during the pregnancy can antagonise the effect of fludrocortisone leading to dizziness, and an increased dose of fludrocortisone is often needed in the last 3 months. Small increases in hydrocortisone may sometimes be needed during the last few months too.

Extra medication in the form of at least one hydrocortisone injection is needed for childbirth; this is detailed in the surgical guidelines available at **www.addisonsdisease.org.uk**, which covers both normal vaginal and Caesarean births.

If you need to have forceps or an assisted delivery, an additional 24 hrs of hydrocortisone injections may be necessary, depending on how quickly you recover. Similarly, if you have a Caesarean section, you will need an injection of hydrocortisone at the start of the procedure and you should take double doses for 48 hrs afterwards until you are back on your feet.

Genetics

The commonest form of Addison's disease in adults is autoimmune, and this has a genetic basis. It is caused by susceptibility variants in several different genes which together give rise to the tendency to develop Addison's disease.[8]

About one in 50 people with adult-onset autoimmune Addison's disease will have a close relative with the condition, so if you are a parent, the risk of Addison's in each of your children is around 2%. However, those autoimmune disease susceptibility variants also predispose to thyroid problems, type 1 diabetes and several other autoimmune conditions like coeliac disease. So around 20% of people with Addison's will have a relative with thyroid problems, and there may be other family members with different autoimmune problems like rheumatoid arthritis, pernicious anaemia (vitamin B12 deficiency) or the depigmenting skin disease, vitiligo.

In contrast to the adult form of autoimmune Addison's disease, there is a much rarer version of the disease that starts in childhood or teenage years. It affects only 2 or 3 people per million in the UK, but is commoner in Scandinavia. Young people with this condition (called autoimmune polyglandular syndrome type 1; APS1 or APECED) may also have a low blood calcium (hypoparathyroidism), a tendency to get thrush infections (candidiasis), defective teeth enamel and poorly formed finger nails.

Typically, children with this problem have been ill with different things including failure to gain weight and slow growth for much of their lives. This problem is caused by a defective single gene (called AIRE) and you need 2 bad copies to get APS1, giving a risk to brothers and sisters of 25%. A blood test for interferon antibodies is diagnostic for this problem.

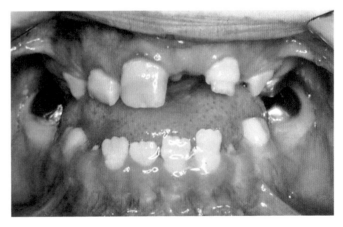

Teeth enamel hypoplasia in a child with APS1/APECED.

What About Sport and Exercise?

Once you have recovered from your pre-diagnosis illness, you can attain a normal level of physical fitness (unless you have other health complications). Everyone benefits from exercising regularly and people with Addison's are no exception to this.

Gentle exercise such as walking and recreational swimming does not usually need extra medication. More physically challenging exercise may mean that you need to take a small extra dose of medication and you should discuss this with your endocrinologist beforehand. The general principle is that if you are used to regularly doing a particular sport or workout, then you probably won't need extra medication. However, if you try a new vigorous workout, take part in a competition or race, then you should generally take a little extra.

For any sports with a risk of physical injury, you should ensure that a team-mate has been trained to administer an emergency injection if needed. This is particularly important if the sport is in a remote location, such as skiing, rock climbing etc.

People with Addison's can (and do) run marathons and take part in other endurance sports, including travelling to remote parts of the world, so it is perfectly possible to realise your ambitions with the right level of support.

Please remember it is important to make sure you stay well hydrated and you should not consume sports drinks with high potassium content, as if you become dehydrated or salt (sodium) depleted, then high blood potassium can be a particular problem for people with Addison's.

Signs of Over and Under Medication

Although it is tempting to think that more medication will always make you feel better, this isn't necessarily true. There is a big difference between taking an extra few doses of steroid to combat a short-term illness, which will not harm you and is necessary to keep you well, and a daily slight over-replacement with steroid for many years, which might lead to complications.

People who have too low a dose of their steroid medication will tend to feel fatigue or low energy, with poor appetite, nausea or salt-craving and gradual weight loss. In addition, increasing skin pigmentation, low blood pressure or low blood sodium also indicate that more medication is needed.

In contrast, weight gain, foot or ankle swelling, high blood pressure, recurrent infections, easy bruising and insomnia can each suggest overtreatment, and that a reduction in steroid dose would be beneficial. Weight gain due to steroid medication typically tends to go on around your middle, face and neck with a 'moon-face and double-chin' pattern.

Chronic exposure to steroids can cause type 2 diabetes. Information about the development of type 2 diabetes or pre-diabetes can come from a blood test called glycosylated haemoglobin (also known as HbA1c): an increased HbA1c is a good reason to look carefully at your steroid doses, to see if it could be reduced.

Children and Young Adults With Addison's

Addison's is most commonly detected in adults between 30 – 50 years old, and is rare in children.

Where Addison's occurs in children and teenagers, the cause is usually autoimmune destruction. Several different rare conditions can also lead to defective steroid production from birth or early childhood, the commonest of which is called congenital adrenal hyperplasia (CAH).

Some children may become adrenally insufficient (dependent on replacement steroid medication) as a result of the medical treatment they need for severe asthma or other medical conditions, such as pituitary tumours or rare childhood cancers. These children may be taking an alternative drug therapy regimen to the standard hydrocortisone and fludrocortisone treatment, such as prednisolone. In addition, there may be several different hormone replacements or other medications for their underlying health problems.

The hydrocortisone dosage needs more regular monitoring in children than in adults, as doses that are too high may result in slower growth. Furthermore, a child's growth in itself results in a moving target, and it is expected that medication doses will gradually increase as the child increases in size.

Just as for adults, 'little and often' hydrocortisone doses are best. Some children feel well taking 2 or 3 daily doses, but sometimes 4 or even 5 small doses are required if they are to feel at their best. This can be a balance between well-being and practicality. Children are often very active and sometimes higher doses of fludrocortisone than those used in adults may be needed. Salt (sodium chloride) supplements may also be needed - for example in early life. Paediatric specialists will monitor a child's condition or conditions until the child reaches 16 years old, after which there should be a managed transition to adult services.

It may take a child some time to return to good health and fitness, as they may have been very poorly prior to diagnosis, and their body will need to recover and adjust to the medication. These children may have lost muscle strength and at first will be easily tired by normal physical education or games activities. This can be an anxious time for families as they learn how to take responsibility for day-to-day medication adjustments that may be needed.

Children and teenagers often do not recognise when their health is deteriorating, and may not report warning signs of illness or insufficient medication. It is therefore important that those involved in the child's care including school staff are alert to warning signs. It may also be particularly difficult for them to remember to take their lunchtime medication, or to agree to take it in front of their classmates. For young adults, prednisolone may be a useful alternative to hydrocortisone in these circumstances as it may only need to be taken once a day. It is also important that young people with Addison's remember drink appropriate fluids, especially when taking part in sport.

Older children should carry an up to date emergency kit with them at all times. However, at primary school age this should be kept in the classroom or school medical kit and the school first-aider, form teacher or classroom assistant invited to watch injection videos or to attend training.

An Individual Health Plan which will be drawn up for your child or teenager will play a key role in helping them to become skilled at self-management. As your child grows, 3 to 6 monthly regular reviews will monitor their need for increased steroid medications.

More detailed information on supporting a child or teenager with Addison's can be found at **www.addisonsdisease.org.uk**.

Oestrogens, Contraception and Menopause

Women with Addison's disease are allowed to take oestrogen hormone replacement therapy (HRT) after the menopause, and such treatment may reduce the risks of bone loss and future osteoporosis to an extent. Nevertheless, the usual cautions to avoid HRT still apply if you have a heightened risk for breast or gynaecological cancer, or thrombosis.

Oestrogen treatment, including the combined contraceptive pill or menopause hormone replacements, leads to increased binding capacity for cortisol in the blood. This means that both healthy women and those with Addison's disease tend to have higher measurements of blood cortisol when they are taking these medications. Do remind your endocrinologist if you are taking such medication, as this is an important factor in interpreting your blood test results.

Similarly, blood cortisol levels appear higher than expected during pregnancy, as oestrogen levels are also higher. In contrast, after the menopause when oestrogen levels are lower, you blood cannot bind as much cortisol and the blood levels may drop. However, this doesn't mean you need extra medication, as the free cortisol in your blood that is available to your tissues should remain about the same.

Getting Older With Addison's

As you become older, many people become less active. This means that you sweat less and lose less salt from your body, so fludrocortisone doses may need to be reduced. High blood pressure (hypertension) may also occur as you get older. In this situation it is important to look at your fludrocortisone dose, with measurement of blood U&E and renin, as reducing the dose could improve your blood pressure. However, it is important not to stop taking fludrocortisone without monitoring: if you have primary adrenal insufficiency or Addison's disease this could result in adrenal crisis. In general, it is safe to reduce the dose of fludrocortisone to 50 micrograms daily but you should do this under supervision from your endocrinologist. If your blood pressure is still high, a medication that increases the capacity of your blood vessels (a 'vasodilator'), such as a calcium channel blocker (amlodipine, lercanidipine) or an ACE-inhibitor (lisinopril, ramipril) is best. You should avoid diuretic medications (bendroflumethazide or indapamide), as these cause salt loss and could lead to dehydration or adrenal crisis.

Fragile bones, osteoporosis and fractures become more common as you grow older. Even if there are no other risk factors (such as a parent with osteoporosis), all people who have been on replacement steroid doses for more than 10 years should have regular bone density (DEXA) scans. This is particularly important once you reach the age of menopause for women and your 60s for men. If the bone density scan is normal, then it is still a good idea to repeat it every 5 years. If it is abnormal, you may be prescribed a weekly bone-strengthening treatment called a bisphosphonate tablet (alendronic acid or risedronate). If you have an abnormal bone density scan, either on the borderline or after you have started some treatment, you should have the scan repeated more frequently.

Appendix A: References

1. Bleicken B, Hahner S, Ventz M, Quinkler M. Delayed diagnosis of adrenal insufficiency is common: a cross-sectional study in 216 patients. Am J Med Sci. 2010; 339(6): 525-31.

2. British National Formulary BNF [online version Nov 6th 2018: bnf.nice.org.uk]

3. Napier C, Pearce SH. Current and emerging therapies for Addison's disease. Curr Opin Endocrinol Diabetes Obes. 2014;21:147-53.

4. Oksnes M, Björnsdottir S, Isaksson M, Methlie P, Carlsen S, Nilsen RM, Broman JE, Triebner K, Kämpe O, Hulting AL, Bensing S, Husebye ES, Løvås K. Continuous subcutaneous hydrocortisone infusion versus oral hydrocortisone replacement for treatment of Addison's disease: a randomized clinical trial. J Clin Endocrinol Metab. 2014;99:1665-74.

5. Gurnell EM, Hunt PJ, Curran SE, Conway CL, Pullenayegum EM, Huppert FA, Compston JE, Herbert J, Chatterjee VK. Long-term DHEA replacement in primary adrenal insufficiency: a randomized, controlled trial. J Clin Endocrinol Metab 2008; 93:400-9.

6. Wass JA, Arlt W. How to avoid precipitating an acute adrenal crisis. BMJ 2012; 345: e6333

7. Lebbe M, Arlt W. What is the best diagnostic and therapeutic management strategy for an Addison patient during pregnancy? Clin Endocrinol (Oxf). 2013;78:497-502.

8. Mitchell AL, Pearce SH. Autoimmune Addison disease: pathophysiology and genetic complexity. Nat Rev Endocrinol 2012;8:306-16.

Appendix B:
European Patient Support Groups

There are several patient support groups in Europe, which may prove helpful if travelling to or spending time in their country.

United Kingdom
Addison's Disease Self-Help Group
Email: enquiries@addisons.org.uk
Website : www.addisonsdisease.org.uk &
www.addisons.org.uk

Czech Republic - ADDISONICI
Website : addisonici.webnode.cz

Denmark - Addison Foreningen i Danmark
Website : www.addison.dk

Finland - Apeced and Addison association (Apeced ja Addison ry)
Website : www.apeced.org

France - L'Association Surrénales
Website : www.surrenales.com

Germany - Netzwerk Hypophysen- und Nebennierenerkrankungen e.V.

Website : www.glandula-online.de

Iceland - Iceland Addison's Samtökin

Website : https://www.facebook.com/Addisons-Samt%C3%B6kin-194639964623370

Italy - Associazione Italiana Pazienti Addison A.I.P.Ad.

Website : www.morbodiaddison.org

Netherlands - BijnierNET/AdrenalNET

Website : www.bijniernet.nl

Netherlands - Dutch Adrenal Patient Society NVACP

Website : bijniervereniging-nvacp.nl

Norway - Morbus Addison Forening Norge

Website : www.addison.no

Spain - Adisen – Asociación Nacional de Addison y Otras Enfermedades Endocrinas

Website : www.adisen.es

Sweden - Svenska Addisonföreningen

Website : www.addison.se

Switzerland - Wegweiser — Schweizer Selbsthilfegruppe für Krankheiten der Hypophyse und Nebennieren

Website : **www.shg-wegweiser.ch**

Turkey — Addison's Turkey

Website : www.addisonturkiye.com

Appendix C:
Worldwide Patient Support Groups

There are several patient support groups located outside Europe, which may prove helpful if travelling to or spending time in their country.

Africa

South African Addison's Group Support (SAAGS)

P.O.Box 34704,

Newton Park,

6055.

South Africa

Australia

Australian Addison's Disease Association

Website : addisons.org.au

Canada

The Canadian Addison Society

Email: info@addisonsociety.ca

Website : www.addisonsociety.ca

Latin America

Adisen – Asociación Nacional de Addison y Otras Enfermedades Endocrinas

Website : www.adisen.es

United States of America

Adrenal Insufficiency United (AIU)

Email: contact@aiunited.org

Website : aiunited.org

National Adrenal Diseases Foundation

Email: nadfsupport@nadf.us

Website : www.nadf.us

Appendix D:
Additional Steroid Dependence
Patient Support Groups

These groups provide support for autoimmune conditions & other forms of steroid dependence associated with Addison's Disease.

Achalasia Research UK
Website : http://www.achalasiaresearch.uk/

Alopecia UK
Website : http://www.alopeciaonline.org.uk/

ALD Life (Adrenoleukodystrophy (ALD) and adrenomyeloneuropathy (AMN))
Website : http://www.aldlife.org/

AMEND - Association for Multiple Endocrine Neoplasia Disorders)
Website : http://www.amend.org.uk/

Asthma UK
Website : http://www.asthma.org.uk/

British Sjogren's Syndrome Association
Website : http://www.bssa.uk.net/

British Thyroid Foundation
Website : http://www.btf-thyroid.org/

Coeliac UK
Website : https://www.coeliac.org.uk/home/

Crohn's and Colitis UK
Website : http://www.crohnsandcolitis.org.uk/

Diabetes UK
Website : http://www.diabetes.org.uk/

Hypopara UK (Parathyroid)
Website : http://hypopara.org.uk/

Living with CAH (Congenital adrenal hyperplasia)
Website : http://www.livingwithcah.com/cah_types.html

National Rheumatoid Arthritis Society
Website : http://www.nras.org.uk/

Pernicious Anaemia Society
Website : http://www.pernicious-anaemia-society.org/

The Pituitary Foundation
Website : http://www.pituitary.org.uk/

The Vitiligo Society
Website : http://www.vitiligosociety.org.uk/

Appendix E:
Recognising the Signs of
Adrenal Crisis

Adrenal Crisis: Danger Signs

► Extreme weakness, feeling terrible, vomiting, headache

► Light-headedness or dizziness on sitting up or standing up

► Feeling very cold, uncontrollable shaking; back, limb or abdominal pain

► Confusion, drowsiness, loss of consciousness.

⊗ **If this happens, inject yourself with your hydrocortisone ampoule (100mg) and call 999, stating "Addisonian crisis"**

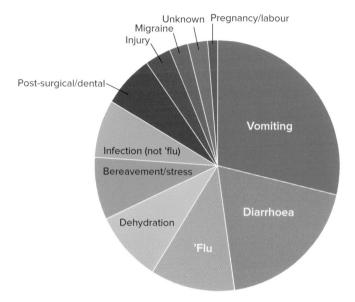

Many things can trigger an adrenal crisis. Learn the risk factors to stay safe.

Appendix F:
Avoiding Adrenal Crisis:
Sick Day Rules

⊗ **You should double your daily hydrocortisone or prednisolone dose if:**

- ▶ You get an infection with a temperature of 38.0°C or higher

- ▶ You get a bad cold, 'flu, diarrhoea or other infection that makes you feel poorly or weak

- ▶ You break a bone or suffer from any similar significant injury

⊗ **Minimum doses**

- ▶ If you take less than 20mg of hydrocortisone in total as your regular daily dose, go up to 40mg daily as a minimum hydrocortisone dose during stress and illness.

- ▶ (*For prednisolone users*) If you take less than 5mg of prednisolone in total as your regular daily dose, go up to 10mg daily as a minimum prednisolone dose during stress and illness.

⊗ **Duration**

- ▶ Keep your dose of steroids doubled for 2 days and then go back to your usual dose, provided that you now feel better.

▶ If you don't feel better after 48hrs, keep your steroid dose doubled and seek advice from your GP or your endocrine nurse or doctor.

▶ If you are prescribed antibiotics for an infection, double your hydrocortisone dose until you finish the course, or feel completely back to normal.

⊗ **Becoming more ill**

▶ If you get a severe infection with a temperature above 40.0°C, then you need to take 3 times your normal hydrocortisone dose and seek advice from your doctor immediately. This could be the start of an adrenal crisis.

▶ If you vomit back your medication within 30 minutes of taking it, take a double dose again immediately. If you vomit this second dose back, then inject yourself with 100mg of hydrocortisone and seek advice. If you carry on vomiting, you will become dehydrated and this will develop into an adrenal crisis unless you go to hospital for a saline drip.

Printed in Great Britain
by Amazon